what's your excuse
for not getting fit

what's your excuse ...

FOR NOT

GETTING FIT?

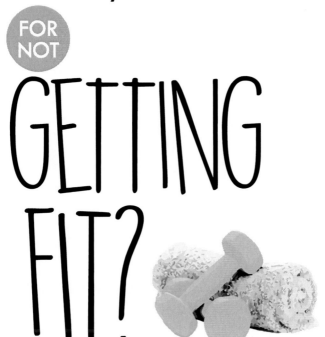

**Overcome your excuses and get
active, healthy and happy**

Waterford City and County
Libraries

joanne henson

"Joanne is a true inspiration! Her passion, commitment and no nonsense attitude never fails to motivate her clients to get moving and achieve their health and fitness goals"

Sarah Price, triathlete and five times Ironman finisher

"Very useful, very readable, and full of sensible, practical advice – that actually makes sense. If you're struggling to keep to an exercise plan, then this will really help"

Chantal Cooke, award winning journalist & broadcaster

"For every excuse, Joanne gives well thought through, sensible solutions which kick your particular excuse into touch. When you see the sense of her arguments, it helps you to really look at what is stopping you from exercising"

Deborah Henry-Pollard, Catching Fireworks

"This book makes you realise you are not a freak for finding reasons not to get up and do it. And it helped me get past those reasons, laugh at myself a little and then come up with strategies that might actually work. A great book to dip in and out of – just reading the contents page is enough to make me smile. Thanks!"

Jan Doole, Business Coach

"You'd probably expect the tone of the book to be shouty and aggressive but surprisingly, it isn't. It has a tone of empathy combined with realism, a kind of 'I understand but come now it is possible'"

beyondthebathroomscale.co.uk

"It's like you're having a conversation with one of those people who doesn't take any of your shit. Reading these books is like someone holding up a big mirror to your whining, excuse-making, sorry self. Joanne has an answer for every excuse, so you're left with '… er… ok. I'll join the gym and buy some apples'. And then… the books sit there and taunt you… There's nothing in these books that's ground breaking but that's the beauty of them. They tell you everything you already knew, in language you can understand. They're like that voice in your head that's usually drowned out by your expert excuse-maker voice. And yeah, after reading these books I got up off my behind and joined the gym"

singlemotherahoy.com

What's Your Excuse for not Getting Fit?

First published in 2013 by Completely Novel
This new edition published in 2015 by WYE Publishing
9 Evelyn Gardens, Richmond TW9 2PL
www.wyepublishing.com

ISBN 978-0-9933388-0-9

Cover and text design by Annette Peppis & Associates

Printed in UK by Marston Book Services Ltd, Oxfordshire

'What's Your Excuse…?' is a UK Registered Trade Mark
(Registration No: 3018995)

www.whatsyourexcuse.co.uk
Follow What's Your Excuse…? on Twitter – @whats_yr_excuse

www.joannehenson.co.uk
Follow Joanne on Twitter – @joannemh

Contents

Introduction

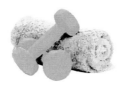

How to use this book

If you've ever embarked on a plan to get fit and healthy, you'll know that the journey is not straightforward. You'll experience periods of high motivation, but these will be interspersed with times when you just can't seem to get your trainers on, or when life seems to get in the way.

I'll say right now that this book is not a new "get fit quick" plan – I am not going to tell you what to do, nor how to do it. What I do in this book is help you to look at the obstacles to your fitness ambitions from new angles. If you are currently finding excuses to skip exercise and you're not getting the results you want, your approach needs an overhaul, and this is where examining the excuses you use will help.

During my many years' involvement in fitness and healthy eating I have heard the same excuses for not sticking to health and fitness resolutions over and over again. I used to use some of these excuses myself. What I've compiled here is a collection of every excuse I have ever heard, with ideas and suggestions on how to overcome them. When you've read my suggestions, you might have some ideas of your own – it's all about creative thinking.

You can use this book in several ways:

If you actually don't really want to get fit and you enjoy your sedentary lifestyle, I'm giving you a source of new excuses to remain just the way you are! The next time someone asks you to go for a run with them, or join them for a game of tennis, or to try a new class at the gym, grab this book, have a quick look at the contents page, and there's bound to be an excuse just ready-made for the moment. In fact, just rip out the contents page and carry it around with you as a handy cheat sheet! You won't need to read the rest of the book.

Seriously though, I'm assuming that if you've bought this book you genuinely want to improve your level of fitness and that you are looking for motivation and support in your endeavours. This book is for you.

You may want to read this book from cover to cover to absorb its positive messages and kick-start a new drive towards getting fit. If so, it will certainly help strengthen your resolve. You should definitely read the introductory chapters to set the scene.

But this book is also designed as a handy reference guide and quick fix for those moments when you find yourself at risk of not getting to the gym, getting on your bike or doing your home workout. When you feel an excuse coming on, look it up and read the tips on how to tackle what's going on in your head. The purpose of each chapter is to help you set aside your excuse, stay focused and continue your journey towards a healthier, fitter you.

Be aware that I'm not offering miracle solutions here – getting fit requires effort. But if you truly want to get fitter I'm offering new ways of thinking about your motivation, your approach and your beliefs about yourself so that you can develop a more positive relationship with exercise.

And if you find yourself coming up with innovative and creative excuses which do not appear in this book, I would love to hear from you – I will incorporate them into the next edition!

Finally, if you are struggling with your diet too, look out for my book *"What's Your Excuse for not Eating Healthily?"*

The benefits of being fit and healthy

Before you move on to the excuses, it's worth reminding yourself of your reasons for wanting to get fit in the first place.

Research shows over and over again that when you have a goal, the more you remind yourself of its benefits, and the more you visualise how it will feel when you get there, the more inspired you will be to continue to work towards it.

So find a notepad and take a few minutes to jot down the reasons why you want to get fit. This will be your own personal Benefits List.

If you're stuck, here are some ideas:

- I won't struggle to run for buses
- I will feel and look better in my clothes
- I will feel and look better naked
- I'll be better able to play with the kids
- I won't have to shop in plus size stores
- My health problems will improve and I may be able to reduce my medication
- I'll be better in bed
- I will feel great

- I might live longer
- I will have more energy
- My skin will glow
- I'll be signing up for the Race for Life/10k/half or full marathon
- I'll be getting complements on how good I look
- I won't have bingo wings/a muffin top
- I'll prove all those people wrong who said I couldn't do it
- I will no longer consider myself lazy
- I'll be picked for the football/netball/cricket team
- I'll have abs instead of a belly
- I'll be enjoying bike rides/long walks/tennis games with my partner/ friends/family
- I may be able to eat more
- I will have grown mentally as well as physically
- I will have mastered a new sport
- I'll know that I am in the best shape of my life
- I'll know that I have overcome my excuses!

From now on, whenever you find yourself about to use an excuse to avoid a workout, take a look at your Benefits List to remind you of your ultimate goal, and of how the new, fitter, healthier you will feel if you set that excuse to one side.

The consequences of not being fit

The previous chapter was intended to emphasise how life can be so much better when you're fit and well.

You might also want to remember how being unfit can adversely affect your life, beyond the obvious visible signs such as being overweight or looking out of shape.

A lack of physical activity means you're not prepared for some of the fun stuff in life, such as a walk along a picturesque coastline on holiday, a kick-about in the park, the Mums' race at your child's school sports day or getting to the top of a hill to admire the view. What should be enjoyable turns into an uncomfortable struggle.

Mood swings, insomnia and low energy levels can also be caused by a lack of exercise, and hidden conditions such as high blood pressure, diabetes and heart disease are linked to low levels of fitness.

Any increase in your activity level is going to decrease your chances of suffering from a wide range of mental and physical problems.

The definition of fitness

Fitness means different things to different people. Your own definition is likely to be contained in your Benefits List, and it could be very different to other readers' definitions. It could also be dictated by the activities you like most, your lifestyle, your age, any medical conditions, your current level of fitness and even your friends. And that's absolutely fine. The purpose of this book is to help motivate you to reach your own personal fitness goals, whatever they may be; it's not a prescription for specific exercises.

But for reference here are all of the key components of all-round fitness, and how to improve them:

Muscular Strength
The ability of your muscles to lift, carry or push against heavy loads. To increase strength you need to train with relatively heavy resistance (eg. weights, resistance bands) for a low number of repetitions.

Muscular Endurance
While strength is a measure of how much force your muscles can exert, endurance is about how many times

your muscles can repeat a move. Improving your muscular endurance requires higher repetitions with less resistance, such as the moves in a Body Pump class, where you work with a weighted bar for the duration of the class.

Cardiovascular Fitness

The ability of your heart, lungs and blood vessels to pump oxygen to your muscles to keep you moving. It's sometimes referred to as Stamina, and it's all about you being able to keep going for prolonged periods of time. Activities such as running, swimming, group fitness classes and cycling will improve your cardiovascular fitness.

Flexibility

The ability of your body to move through its entire range of motion. This element of fitness is often overlooked but a lack of flexibility in certain parts of your body can lead to imbalances in others, and can prevent you from performing exercises correctly. Imbalances and badly performed exercises cause injury, so it's well worth including some mobility exercises into your routine, as it will improve your performance in everything else and reduce the risk of injury. Stretching, yoga, foam rolling and massages all contribute to better flexibility.

Body Composition

This element of fitness is the most easily misunderstood. It's all about not carrying too much body fat in proportion to lean tissue (muscle, bones, skin, water, etc) but all too often it's over simplified: Thin is deemed to be fit and Fat is deemed to be unfit. In fact it's perfectly possible to look thin but have poor body composition, or to look fatter but have good body composition, as it's about the *ratio* of fat to other tissue, not just overall weight or lack of visible fat. So just because you're thin it doesn't mean that you've got this element covered – you need to have a healthy amount of lean tissue to fat, and that's best achieved by incorporating resistance training into your regime.

In addition to the main elements of fitness there are other skill-related elements: agility, balance, speed, reaction time, power and coordination. These are generally more relevant to sports than to general fitness activities, but it's worth being aware of these as you may find that as you get fitter or participate in a wider range of activities these skills will improve of their own accord, and if they do you should acknowledge that and be proud of the improvement.

If any of this information has given you new ideas or a better understanding of how fitness will feel, you might want to add what you have learnt to your Benefits List before continuing.

The Excuses

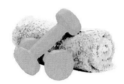

An excuse becomes an obstacle in your journey to success when it is made in place of your best effort or when it is used as the object of the blame.

Bo Bennett

Obstacles don't have to stop you. If you run into a wall, don't turn around and give up. Figure out how to climb it, go through it, or work around it.

Michael Jordan

Mind

I hate the gym/exercise

All gyms and *all* exercise? Have you tried every gym in your area and every sport/activity you can think of?

There are always going to be activities which some people enjoy more than others. I hate running, but love weight training. My next door neighbours run every day, but I am pretty sure they never set foot in a gym. Some people like team sports, others like more solitary pursuits. We are all different. So if you've only tried the obvious, try something new.

What is it you hate about the gym or whatever else you've tried? What does your chosen form of exercise absolutely not have to include? Try to write down what you dislike and what you find more bearable. Do you like exercising with a friend or do you need to exercise alone? Do you like being outdoors, or do you hate being cold and wet? Do you need variety or do you like the familiar?

Of course all things worth having have to be earned, and fitness is no different – you've got to put the effort in. But at the same time you should be able to identify forms of exercise which are more appealing than others.

Here are some ideas to get you started:

Weight training	Salsa
Running	Belly dancing
Swimming	Tennis
Pilates	Cycling
Yoga	Step class
Climbing	Body combat
Gymnastics	Martial arts
Kettlebells	Body pump
CrossFit	Ballet
Walking/hiking	Creative dance
Rowing	Zumba
Athletics	Boxing
Football	Personal training
Netball	Boot camp
Basketball	Squash
Ballroom dancing	

Try a few new forms of exercise, ideally a whole lot of different things. There's bound to be something you find more fun, satisfying and/or motivating than what you've tried before.

I've got no willpower

Are there times when you are so driven that nothing will stop you getting to the gym? What's different about those times, and this time?

The answer is likely to be the level of focus you have – when you feel like you've got willpower in spades it's because your end goal is at the forefront of your mind. You want the end result so much that you're willing to put the effort in to get there. So if you made a Benefits List as I suggested at the beginning of this book, take a look at it. There's a saying, "Begin with the end in mind" but I think it's more about *progressing* with the end in mind. Remind yourself *all the time* why you are doing this.

There are lots of ways of keeping your mind on the prize. Consider making a vision board for instance, with images of what you are working towards and what it might look like – finishing a race, scoring a goal or simply looking fitter.

Also, surround yourself with positive people, and with people who have similar goals to you. This is why the experience of being in a gym works so well for some people, me included. When you're surrounded by other people all working to improve their own strength/stamina/flexibility/coordination, it's inspiring. Whereas if you're surrounded by people complaining about how boring exercise is and how you really ought to give the gym a miss and go to the pub... well, what do you think might happen?

However, by far the best way to tackle wavering willpower is to reduce the need for it as much as possible. In his book "Happiness by Design", Paul Dolan talks about setting default options for yourself. He says that the average human being is pretty lazy and is generally predisposed to go with the flow, or do

> Remind yourself *all the time* why you are doing this.

whatever is easiest. So if you make it as easy as possible to choose the gym over the sofa, you're setting a default option which you'll end up doing because it's not an effort.

How do you do this? You get home from work, you were planning to go to a group fitness class at the gym, but you're tired and you need to get your kit together and the sofa is calling... wouldn't it be an easier decision to make if you had arranged to meet a friend at the class, or if you had a personal trainer waiting for you at the gym? If you had paid up front or booked in? If you had your gym bag packed and ready to go by the door? If you joined a gym which was on your way home from work rather than a car ride away in the opposite direction?

Don't leave yourself in a position where you have to rely solely on willpower to get your running kit on or get to the gym – make it easy for yourself by better organising your situation.

I'm not in the mood

There are lots of things you do regularly for which you're never in the mood – going to the dentist, taking the car for a service, picking up the dog's poo, even going to work every morning. So you don't actually have to be in the mood in order to do anything.

What you *are* in the mood for is improving your health, and all the benefits you know that improved health will bring.

So in the words of a famous sports clothing company, *just do it*.

See also "I can't get motivated".

I don't want to look stupid

No one does, and writing as someone who has stepped the wrong way in group fitness classes more times than

I care to remember, I know what it's like to feel stupid when exercising.

But other people are a lot less interested in your mistakes than you imagine. Regular gym goers really aren't wasting their time looking out for beginners to ridicule – they are busy with their own workout, or concentrating on getting their own moves right. And *everyone* has to concentrate in a class – no one knows the moves so well that they can switch to auto-pilot.

Should you come across people who do try to make you feel bad, consider this – they're most likely doing it to feel better about themselves. They're not happy in their own skin, their behaviour is not about you and if you weren't around they'd find someone else.

It's about being the best *you* can be, not *the* best.

You can't change the behaviour of other people, but you can change your reaction to them. So don't take it personally, give them a smile (that will irritate them!) and move along.

Getting fit is all about improving *your* fitness, not competing with everyone else. Learn to congratulate yourself for progress made, and for being fitter than you were last week or last month or last year. It's about being the best *you* can be, not *the* best. Which means that if you do slip up in a class or find yourself running on a treadmill more slowly than the person next to you,

you can still be proud that you're there, doing it and improving.

I'm too stressed

Extreme stress is horrible. It saps your energy, mentally and physically, and seeps into every waking moment. Yes, I've been there, and even though I knew that getting fitter and healthier would help with my stress levels, I wasn't in a position to act on that knowledge because all of my mental energy was used up in dealing with the stress. But extreme stress is something you won't be able to tolerate forever – something will eventually give, and it's best if it's not you. What is more important – the source of your stress or your own health?

If you are very stressed it's likely that the source of your stress is either work or relationship/family related – so I appreciate that it's not likely to be something you can simply walk away from. If that's the case, to survive with your health intact you need change your response to it. Ask yourself whether it's worth the expenditure of your emotional energy. Ask yourself if the damage it is doing to your health is worth it. And ask yourself if feeling stressed is actually productive – it's generally not, and it generally doesn't help a situation.

Once you come to see the stress for the waste of time and energy it is, you are in a better position to start making changes – however small.   Start reading up on stress relief strategies – "Stress Proof Your Life" by Elisabeth Wilson gives simple and practical tips for dealing with your situation. Not all of them will work for you, but if just a handful do, it's progress.

Be kind to yourself and take care of your body.

Exercise is a fantastic antidote to stress – it can control current physical and emotional effects and helps our bodies and minds become more resilient for future stress. Some studies have shown that exercise can be as effective as anti-depressants. But if you're so overwhelmed with stress that you're not exercising at all at the moment, take baby steps towards looking after your health by introducing some pleasure into your life. You might not be able to face a workout, but start scheduling treat time into your diary – go for a massage, get to the cinema or theatre, eat out, visit or just call a friend. Think of pleasure as a nutrient that will counteract what stress is doing to your body.

Then, once you've got into the habit of taking time out for yourself, start scheduling in some exercise, and if necessary some time to plan healthy meals, to replace the vitamins and minerals which stress depletes. Take it slowly, but be kind to yourself and take care of your body – it's the only one you'll ever have and it's not worth sacrificing it to a stressful job or relationship.

Now, if when you say you're too stressed you really mean you've had a bad day or bad week and just need to kick back and have a couple of glasses of wine in front of the TV rather than go to your yoga class, then tell me – is it a one-off? If it is, it's not the end of the world if you give yourself a break. But if this is a regular thing for you, then once again you need to tackle the stress and re-prioritise your health – go back to the paragraphs above.

I'm bored with my workout

I suspect that everyone gets bored with their workouts from time to time – so what to do? Hmmm, let me think…..... how about *changing your workout*?

Try something new, or just take a new approach to your current favourite exercise. If you cycle or run, find a new route, or travel the same route in reverse. If you work out with weights, change your routine, if you usually do Body Pump, do a spin class. Learn to climb or go to a boot camp – the possibilities for change are endless.

The fact is, if you are bored by your workout your body is probably bored too, so it will stop responding and improving. So being bored is good – it's a prompt to do something different, try a new challenge. You might even find yourself going back to your old workout with renewed enthusiasm once you've had a break.

I can't get motivated

It's great when you feel all fired up about your workout and can't wait to get into the gym/the pool/your running shoes. But there are bound to be times when you don't feel quite so enthusiastic – you're tired, there's something interesting on the TV, or you just don't feel like it (see also "I'm not in the mood").

If you think about other areas of your life, I'm sure there are lots of things you do all the time despite not really being motivated to do them. Going to work on a Monday morning, for instance, or cleaning the toilet. Why do you do them? If you don't go to work you'd be in trouble with your boss and you might not get paid, and the result of never cleaning your toilet wouldn't be pleasant. Both of these things you do because you want to avoid the consequences of not doing it, not because you are motivated.

And then there are things you do out of sheer habit, like showering and brushing your teeth – I'm guessing you never get up in the morning and consider whether you need to do these things, you *just do them*. Try to think about exercise as one of these regular maintenance tasks that you just wouldn't dream of neglecting.

But you can also "act as if". If one of my clients says to me "I can't get motivated to go to the gym" I ask her, how would a motivated person behave? They'd go to the gym. I'd then suggest that just once in the following week, my client acts *as if* she is motivated. She doesn't have to *be* motivated, she just has to *act as if* she is. And when you act as if you are motivated for long enough, who needs motivation? You're developing habits that mean you are doing it anyway.

It's no fun

Some forms of exercise are more fun than others – zumba classes, belly dancing, walking and team games (if you're a team player) can all be done with a smile on your face.

But if you are looking to improve your fitness levels, remember this – if you always do what you've always done, you'll always get what you always got. So you are going to have to push your boundaries from time to time, and if you're pushing yourself then no, it's not always going to feel like fun.

Running faster than ever before to complete your usual 10k in 30 seconds less, adding an extra 5kg to your deadlift, challenging a better player to a tennis match – they are all going to stretch you. But that's what improvement is all about – *if it doesn't challenge you it doesn't change you*.

So it's not always fun – but it is energising, stimulating, satisfying, pride-inducing, good for your health, anti-ageing, positive, fulfilling, rewarding, mood-lifting… feel free to add more words of your own. And feeling fit and well can be fun in itself.

Environment

It's raining

I'm writing this in the UK, and assuming that you're probably in the UK too. So you should be used to rain by now – you know, that thing that comes as part and parcel of our British Summers? And our British Springs, Autumns and Winters.

If your fitness plans include outdoor activities you're kidding yourself if you think that you're always going to be exercising on dry days. There are going to be whole weeks when it's pouring down, and if you let the rain put you off, that means there will be whole weeks when you don't exercise.   If you're serious about your outdoor activity, you need to accept that rain comes as part of the deal, and live with it.

If you are reading this because you're really not fancying that run/cycle ride/football match you had planned for today because it's raining outside, have a look at your Benefits List. Remind yourself why you are doing this. And then remind yourself it's only 30/45/60 minutes. And once it's over, how could you reward yourself when you get back? A nice warm shower or bath? And won't that feel great? Going out in the rain might not feel good but getting back into the warm, dry house knowing that you've just ticked off a workout will feel fantastic.

For the future, consider your clothing – do you need better, waterproof kit? Investing in more suitable wet weather clothing could make a difference to how you feel about exercising in the rain.

But if going out in the rain really doesn't do it for you, and you aren't wedded to a specific outdoor activity, why not consider some indoor alternatives so that you have something different up your sleeve for rainy days? How about fitness DVDs, Wii Fit or a trip to the gym to use the treadmill? Buy a DVD, look into pay-as-you-go gyms and do the preparation so you have the alternatives readily organised for when the heavens open.

It's too cold/too hot

There is a saying which goes something like "There's no such thing as the wrong weather, only the wrong clothes". It's been attributed to Billy Connolly but I'm sure he's not the first person to have said this.

Much of what I've said under "It's raining" above is also relevant to this excuse – the climate in most coun-

tries is changeable, and if you've picked an outdoor activity as a means to get fit, you're not going to be doing
it in perfect weather conditions every time.

So if the weather is a constant bugbear for you,
is your chosen activity really the best one for you? Do
you want to continue with it because you enjoy it when
the weather's behaving?
If so, can you live with a
lack of improvement due
to the intermittent nature
of your workouts?   Do
you need to think of an-
other means of exercising
for the days when you don't want to be outside? How
much do you want to get fit and what compromises are
you willing to make?

There's no such thing as the wrong weather, only the wrong clothes.

Finally, I appreciate that sometimes weather conditions can be extreme – icy roads are probably not a
good surface for running or cycling and desert-like heat
is not ideal for endurance sport. But often when I hear
the "It's too cold/too hot" excuse it's not due to extreme
weather conditions, it's generally because today is a few
degrees colder than yesterday (and anyway EastEnders
is about to start), or the sun is shining so brightly that it
feels like the right time to find a beer garden. Is it really
the weather which is putting you off?

Knowledge

I don't know what to do

Nobody does when they start out – did you know how to drive a car when you first got into the driver's seat?

Everyone starts somewhere – Chris Froome would have had to learn to ride a bike as a child and Jessica Ennis would have had plenty of coaching sessions on her way to winning Olympic gold.

There's no shame in being a beginner – you're beginning, which puts you in a better place than all of those people still sat on the sofa. And there is a whole industry of trainers, coaches and YouTube regulars who are reliant on beginners to make a living.

How would you learn something at work or at home? You would ask for help from someone who's done it before, or copy someone, or buy a book and read up about it first. Everyone starts out as a beginner. Don't be afraid to ask for advice from experienced exercisers, or from gym staff. That's what they are there for and your gym membership fee pays their salaries.

I am worried about getting too muscly

I'm assuming you're female if you're reading this, as I have *never* heard this excuse from a man.

So let me put you straight on women and muscles. Women have more oestrogen and less testosterone than men, both of which mean that the growth of large and bulky muscles is inhibited in the female body. So you won't end up looking like a man by following a regular exercise regime. Female bodybuilders achieve their size by training hard and training often, and sometimes by using stuff they shouldn't be using.

As a woman you shouldn't be put off weight training as it offers two real benefits.

One is that the additional lean muscle mass that you do build will increase your metabolism – the more muscle you carry around, the more calories you burn every day. In fact if you are looking to lose body fat, weight training is far more effective than a program of pure cardio, however much you sweat during the cardio.

'Toned' is really just a combination of less body fat and firmer muscles.

And if you've ever said you want to be more toned,

note that "toned" is really just a combination of less body fat and firmer muscles – which regular training with weights will deliver.

The second benefit of resistance training and weight bearing exercise is that it helps improve bone strength and ward off osteoporosis. And the fitter you are as you age the less likely you are to have the sort of falls which cause fractures. So get strong to stay strong.

Finally, you are not going to suddenly wake up one morning looking like Arnie! Muscle growth is very, very gradual. I promise you that muscles are not going to suddenly take you by surprise!

Body

It's too hard

OK, it's true that getting fit is not a piece of cake (I was going to say "walk in the park", but it could be!) If getting and staying fit were easy, we'd be a far more active nation. In fact the act of getting fitter by its very nature involves challenging yourself and pushing boundaries. But if you've made the decision to read this book, I assume you're still set on the challenge, and you now have your Benefits List as a reminder of why it will be worthwhile.

I actually believe there is more than one type of Hard.

The first is the "I didn't realise it would be so difficult" variation of Hard. It is possible, if you're new to exercise or starting exercise again after a long period of inactivity, that you've dived too deep, too quickly into a hard core programme for which your body is not ready and which it therefore really isn't enjoying. Trying too hard too soon is the classic mistake made by a lot of January resolution-makers – diving straight in to something which is way beyond their levels of fitness, so that their workouts are a humiliating struggle. Why would anyone want to stick to something like that?

In her book "The 4-Day Win", Martha Beck talks about "edging into exercise". She quotes a friend of hers who told her, "Ninety percent of being in shape is getting to the gym". He said this to her at a time when she was overweight and not exercising at all, but aware that she needed to change. So in the interests of edging herself into exercise, her first "workouts" were simply getting to the gym – yes, just getting to the gym, but not going in. She drove to the gym every day for four days, parked in the car park, then drove home again. After that, for the next four days, she drove to the gym, went in, and did three minutes of exercise, then drove home again. After that she upped it to seven minutes, and so on. Not long into this very gradual transition into exercise, she found herself wanting to do more than she was planning, and felt like her body had "decided that it actually *loved* the gym".

Trying too hard too soon is the classic mistake.

So gradual can be good. There is absolutely no need to throw yourself into something at an advanced level on day one. Martha upped her commitment every four days – so within a month she would have been doing 20-30 minute workouts, and the advantage was that she ended up actually itching to progress faster. Easing yourself in gently will still get you there in the end, and minimises the chances of you giving up because it all feels too Hard.

The other variation on Hard? "I don't like working so hard". If you find yourself saying this, ask

Seeing results tends to put even the hardest workouts into perspective.

yourself exactly what it is that you find Hard. It might be a case of what I described above, or it might be that you've simply chosen the wrong activity for you. I personally can't stand running – I find it boring, and pushing myself to improve at it just doesn't inspire me, so I find any sort of running Hard. Whereas the effort and focus involved in training with heavy weights doesn't strike me as Hard at all, because I find it really satisfying. So consider the possibility that you're just in the wrong gym class or forcing yourself to persevere with the wrong activity. Do you prefer to exercise with friends, or in a class, or would you prefer to be going it alone? Do you like to be outdoors or indoors? Find something better suited to your preferences and even if it doesn't feel easy, it could feel a lot less Hard.

Also, if you're going to put in the effort, do make sure that what you're doing best serves your goals. Seeing results tends to put even the hardest workouts into perspective, so make sure you're not wasting your time on activities which won't deliver what you want to achieve. For instance, running alone won't give you more muscle definition and pilates won't burn fat). Sounds obvious, but I personally wasted many, many hours of my life doing cardio, hoping it would give me muscle definition. I switched to weight training and – ta da! – I started seeing results and my gym visits seemed a whole lot easier.

I don't have the energy to exercise

Countless studies have found that regular exercise reduces feelings of fatigue. Activity energises, but then you probably already know that.

When you're feeling absolutely knackered – physically, mentally or both – how do you find the energy to put on your kit, never mind to do the workout?

Firstly, consider how energised you'll feel after a workout – even ten minutes is going to be better than nothing at all. You might not have the energy for the 20 mile bike ride you'd planned, but do you have the energy for 5 miles, or even 1 mile? So ask yourself what could you manage? (There's every chance that once you've started your energy levels will rise and you'll end up doing more than the 1 or 5 miles anyway).

If this happens a lot, consider whether you are planning your workouts at the wrong time of day. If you tend to get in from work pretty late, when you're hungry and tired and it's dark outside, is it reasonable to expect yourself to get changed and go out again for a run or drive to the gym? What about exercising at lunchtimes or before work instead?

Don't forget to drink lots of water.

Studies proving that exercise is energising often go on to say that morning workouts are particularly effective. Studies also show that people who exercise early in the day are more likely to stick with their programme than those who exercise at other times of the day. From my experience, morning workouts are least likely to suffer from "something came up". No one's going to ask for you for an impromptu beer at 7.00am, nor is your boss around to ask you to do an extra half hour at the office.

And for the future, think about your eating patterns – if you get home from work at 6.30 and the last meal you had was a sandwich at lunchtime, your energy levels are bound to be depleted – keep a snack at the office and eat it just before you leave, giving it time to get turned into fuel for your workout.

Finally, don't forget to drink lots of water – a dehydrated body is a sluggish and weary body.

I didn't see any changes in my body the last time I exercised

How long did you stick at the exercise last time?

Was the exercise you chose suitable for achieving the results you want?

And if your target was to lose weight did you make any changes to your diet?

In fact, what was your target? *Specifically?* In terms of speed reached, time taken, goals scored, height climbed, lengths swum, etc?

I'm asking you these questions because exercise *does work*, when done consistently over a period of time and when it's appropriate to your goal.

Let's look at time first. Every week I see women's magazines featuring a new "get toned in 4 weeks plan" (and then the "plan" generally includes exercises which really wouldn't challenge any body enough to change it within a year, never mind 4 weeks, but that's a rant I will set aside for another time). If these plans included a pretty strict diet you would see a change in your measurements within 4 weeks, but not a major change in your body shape, nor its tone, unless you are one of the lucky few whose body responds very quickly to exercise. From experience I would say that you have to exercise consistently for 2-3 months before you see real changes. And if you want to make really big changes it will take longer. Sorry if that's not what you want to hear, but being fit is a lifestyle, not a quick fix.

Next up, was the exercise you did last time suitable for the results you were trying to achieve? Do you want to run a 10k race? Then you need to run. Do you want to tone up? Then you shouldn't be running – try a form of resistance training.

On the subject of weight loss, if you are exercising simply to lose weight but you haven't made changes to your diet, you're going to struggle. Serious and long lasting weight loss is more about cleaning up your diet (and I do mean cleaning up the quality of your food and not just reducing the quantity) than it is about exercise.

Although I don't believe that the complicated business of fat loss can be reduced to a calories-in-calories-out computation, I am going to use calories to illustrate this point. It's generally believed that one pound of body fat is the equivalent of around 3,500 calories. On average, it's estimated that men burn 483 calories in a Body Pump class and women burn 338. So according to the calories-in-calories-out theory an average sized woman would have to do over ten Body Pump classes per week to lose one pound of fat through exercise alone. Or she could reduce her calorie consumption by 500 calories per day. 500 calories is one Starbucks Grande White Chocolate Mocha, an average restaurant dessert, a large portion of fries or 5 chocolate biscuits. What sounds easiest? The comparison is overly simplistic,

Exercise is an important element of permanent weight loss.

but it does illustrate how important diet is in maintaining a healthy weight. And I mean having a healthy diet rather than being 'on' a diet.

Having said all of that, exercise is an important element of permanent weight loss as it helps to keep your metabolism fired up and builds all-important muscle fibres which use extra calories all day long. Resistance training is more effective than cardio for this, particularly steady state cardio. If you must do cardio and your goal is weight loss, do intervals. Look up HIIT (High Intensity Interval Training) to learn about how you can adapt your cardio routine to burn more fat.

Finally, you won't be able to judge progress or change if you can't measure it. If you make your fitness goal clear, specific and measurable, you have something against which you can chart your progress. So write down how many inches you want to lose, how quickly you want to run the Race for Life, or how many press ups you want to do. Then track your progress, and write it down *every* time. You may only see small improvements, but those small improvements will add up to one great big one if you stick at it.

For example, say you do your usual run today in fifteen seconds' less time than you did three days ago. If you'd casually glanced at the kitchen clock as you left the house and then casually glanced again when you got back, you probably wouldn't appreciate that there'd been any improvement. But if you bought yourself a stopwatch, or wore a wristband monitor, or used an app on your smart phone to time your run accurately, you'd know about those fifteen seconds. And you'd be more likely to go out again in two days' time to try to knock another fifteen seconds off today's time. Similarly, an inch lost off your waist might not be visible from a glance in the mirror, but a tape measure would record it for you. So get measuring, recording and timing!

I'm worried about overtraining

It *is* possible to overtrain – if you do the same workout over and over again without adequate rest in between. A single activity done repeatedly and too often could put a strain on particular muscles or joints and cause injury over time.

But our bodies, if they are well-nourished and well-rested, can be remarkably resilient. I saw a tweet recently which said, "There's no such thing as over-training, just under-eating and under-sleeping". A bit extreme maybe, but nutrition and rest do have a massive effect on exercise performance and results. If you support regular exercise with good quality food and adequate sleep, you'll be maximising the benefits of your workouts *and* reducing the chances of injury or overtraining.

Support regular exercise with good quality food and adequate sleep.

If you don't feel any aches, pains or soreness anywhere, you're not about to overtrain by doing another workout – so if you find yourself using this as an excuse to have another rest day, whilst not really pushing yourself when you do go to the gym, you're being overly cautious.

If you are sore (and not actually injured) from yesterday's workout, then well done! I'll take that as a sign that your last workout was suitably challenging and effective. And it doesn't hurt to take a day off now and again. But many fitness professionals talk about "active rest", times when they keep their bodies moving but don't push it to the max. This helps keep blood flowing to muscles which are repairing themselves after an intense workout the day before – so even if you do feel a bit sore you can still go for a walk in the park or a swim, or do a stretch class.

It's about exercising consistently, regularly, and effectively.

One final question for you – are you doing three or more *effective* and *varied* workouts a week? If so, you really don't need an excuse to take the other days of the week off. Fitness is not about exercising every day, it's about exercising consistently, regularly, and *effectively*.

It hurts

Hurts? Or just hard work?

For just hard work, see "It's too hard".

But if you are injured you have a valid excuse – temporarily! If you continue to exercise with an injury you'll make it worse, so you really do need to rest. If after a few days rest it's not better, see a health professional – a physiotherapist, an osteopath or another suitably qualified practitioner, and *follow their advice*.

I'm hungover

Now you know you only have yourself to blame for this! And there is not a lot you can do to change a hangover once you've got it (sorry but I don't think full English breakfasts, full sugar Coke, brown toast and honey or strong black coffee actually work).

So, since you can't turn back time to fix the current hangover, let's think about next time instead.

Before I go on, I will say that there are obviously going to be occasions where you've got a big day/night planned, which you *know* are going to result in a hangover – I'm not about to recommend total abstinence. If you've got a big wedding, birthday party or family event planned then go ahead, have a great time, and live with the hangover. Since you'll have put it in your diary well in advance, you've got the opportunity to plan your workouts around it. No problem.

But the type of hangover we are likely to be talking about here is the one when you planned an early morning run before work on a Thursday, but found yourself in the pub after work on the Wednesday evening, where "just the one" turned into a skin-full. Or the Sunday morning spin class which doesn't happen because you started on the shots when you should have been catching the last train home the night before.

What goes through your head when you know

you've got a workout planned tomorrow but some-one is suggesting you go to the pub, or your other half wants to open a bottle of wine? Might it be "I'll just have the one/two?"

When you agreed to the first drink were you actu-ally planning on having four or five? I'm guessing not. So what is your tip-ping point between still caring about doing that

Alcohol will inhibit weight loss and negate any attempt to get fit or build muscle.

workout the next day and caring more about extending the great time you're having with another drink? And how can you prevent yourself reaching it?

The most effective way of ensuring you don't reach it is obvious – don't start drinking in the first place! Ei-ther go to the pub and drink mineral water, or don't go at all. I realise neither of those options sounds like fun but what do you want more? A fit, healthy, attractive body or three hours in a pub with people you've been working with all day anyway and a whole day of feeling rough tomorrow? Don't kid yourself that you'll go and just have the one or two – if you've never managed to before, how likely is it the next time? Accept it just won't happen and plan accordingly. Make a deal with your-self that you will only go to the pub after work once a week, or twice a month – however many days you think you can reasonably miss the gym without scuppering your fitness goals. And have reasons ready for when you're invited and you want to say no – practice them, and make them positive. My own personal experience here is that you'll be challenged less when you speak in a more positive way. For instance, if you say "I'm not drinking at the moment" you'll find yourself questioned and having to justify yourself. If however you say "I'm going to the gym tomorrow and need to feel my best" that's a positive, clearly stated reason which you'll find more readily accepted. One of my clients who was try-ing to lose weight practiced various "stock" answers for challenging situations – "No thanks, I am eating out lat-er", "No thanks, it was lovely but I'm stuffed now and couldn't eat another mouthful", "Not at the moment, I might have one later" – so that she was never caught out when someone encouraged her to have food which didn't fit into her eating plan. Be ready with your own stock of answers.

And if you need further encouragement to stay out of the pub after work, be aware that alcohol will inhibit weight loss and negate any attempt to get fit or build muscle – not just because of the calories, but because it messes with your nutrition, fluid levels and hormones. Not nice, and those effects last for several days after you've had the drink.

I think I may be getting ill

The generally accepted advice here is if your symptoms are above the neck (runny nose, sore throat) and you're not feverish, then you're OK to go and do some gentle exercise. If your symptoms are below the neck (cough, wheezing) or you are feverish, then don't exercise. *Exercising when you have something worse than a head cold can prolong the illness and in some cases make it worse*. So feel free to rest if you are genuinely ill.

If you are just feeling a bit low, see "I don't have the energy to exercise".

I'm too old

In the past week I've read about two truly inspirational people. Doris Long, 101 years old, became the world's oldest abseiler in July 2015, abseiling 94m down the Spinnaker Tower in Portsmouth after setting the record the year before when she turned 100. When she finished she said, "My legs ache like anything and my right arm…and my hair is all sticking out". Charles Eugster, 95 years old, recently broke the World Masters indoor 200m running record, after taking up weight training at 87 because he felt his body was deteriorating after giving up rowing at 85. He's planning on breaking the outdoor record next.

I'm guessing you're not quite that old?

There is a commonly held belief that as we age our bodies let us down; losing muscle, gaining fat and generally malfunctioning. All of that can and does happen, but it happens more rapidly when you're not fit. Regular exercise preserves muscle, keeps your heart healthy, your bones strong and your joints flexible. Some studies suggest it keeps your mind sharper too. So if you want to feel good as you get older, the earlier you start exercising the better.

Regular exercise preserves muscle, keeps your heart healthy, your bones strong and your joints flexible.

But what if you've not exercised for years and you simply feel too old to start now? The key is to start slowly (see "It's too hard" for just how slowly Martha Beck started). Ease yourself into something gentle (eg. walking, swimming, or some simple yoga moves) and aim for very gradual, small improvements. Start out on the basis that anything is better than nothing – even a five minute walk to the local shop is better than five minutes spent watching TV – and build up from there. Once you get used to moving and start feeling more flexible and confident about what your body can do you can progress to other activities.

If you start something at 40, 50 or 60, you may never be as fast or strong as you might have been at 20, but you'll be good for your age, and that's all that matters.

By the way, I'm well placed to comment on this. I've exercised since the age of 20, but not very effectively. At the age of 40 I signed up with a personal trainer and now, approaching 50, I am fitter, stronger, leaner and more co-ordinated than I have ever been. So I know it is possible to get fitter as you age.

I'm too fat

Is it that you are physically too big, or that you are embarrassed about your body?

If you think you are physically too big to go to the gym, or participate in a Zumba class, or go running, what can you do? Can you walk? For how long? Five minutes a day is better than no minutes a day. Can you play tennis on a Wii, or do a beginners' workout DVD? Anything is better than nothing, and you can add an extra couple of minutes or move a bit faster each time – just start somewhere and improve slowly.

If it's about how you feel about exercising in front of

other people – well, you don't need to exercise in public. Find something you can do in private. How about a Wii, YouTube or DVD workout at home? You can also buy all sorts of equipment to use at home or, if you can afford it, you can have a personal trainer come to your home. As you get fitter and lose weight, you can then reconsider venturing outside or into a gym.

See also "I don't want to look stupid" in the Mind section – no one feels comfortable when they first enter a gym, but they'd probably be surprised at just how little interest most of the regulars have in anyone other than themselves and their own workout. *No one will be watching you anyway.*

I'm already thin so I don't need to exercise

It's a common mistake to measure fitness or health by weight alone, and this can mislead slim people into believing that they must be healthy. They might also look at overweight people and automatically consider them to be unhealthy. In reality it is much more complicated than that. You can be slim without being fit or healthy. For instance you could be a slim smoker, or you could be slim because you only consume 1,000 calories a day, but if they are 1,000 calories of fast food and sugary snacks you'll be malnourished.

The term "skinny fat" is common parlance these days, and there's a reason for that – there is a realisation that you can be slim but not have enough lean muscle to make up a healthy body composition.

So just because you're thin doesn't mean you shouldn't exercise. Our bodies are made to be active.

I'm useless at sport

At school, I was always the last to be picked for the team at every sports session, so what I write here comes from experience.

I have very little natural coordination or spatial awareness, which made me unsuited to every single one of the team games we had to play at school. It did nothing for my self-esteem as a teenager. But, looking back, what I lacked was coaching and support. I never had a chance to get better as I had no advice or guidance and I did all I could to avoid any sort of exercise until my early twenties.

I then ended up sharing a house with someone who was heavily into fitness, but it was *fitness* as opposed to sport – she ran and swam religiously. I realised that you could get fit without being sporty, and you could get fit for your own satisfaction, not for other members of a team. Suddenly, fitness made sense. I initially identified activities which didn't require much co-ordination, such as swimming and cardio machines, and then as my fitness levels and confidence increased I gradually tried more challenging things, such as group fitness classes (starting out by standing right at the back, of course). I also started asking for advice from professionals. It still takes me longer than most to learn new moves, but I am far fitter than I ever believed I could be and because I put in the effort I feel have every right to feel prouder of myself than someone who is a "natural". If I can get fit, anyone can.

Having read my story, you'll appreciate that I've experienced embarrassment in the past – going left in the step class when everyone else was going right, taking much longer to master moves than the rest of the class, being one of the last to finish in races (I was slow to learn to drive too). But was anyone really looking and laughing? As a gym "regular" now, I can honestly say that I am not looking out for beginners to ridicule. I am too focused on my own workout and I am pretty sure that everyone else in the gym is equally focused on their own workouts too.

So if you're useless at team sports, so what? That doesn't make you useless at getting fit. Pick something simple to start with (running, swimming, cardio machines, simple weight training routines), get good at that, and then use your new confidence to tackle something slightly more challenging.

Activities

I walk to the station and back every day, isn't that enough?

You tell me if it's enough – what are your fitness goals? Is a short walk ten times a week enough to achieve them? If you've bought this book I'm assuming that you're not happy with your current fitness levels and therefore the walk to the station and back is not serving you well.

So, no, if you want to get fitter, it's probably not enough.

I keep fit running around after the kids

Now it may be true that running round after your kids is physically challenging, but if you want to improve your fitness levels rather than just maintain what you have, you need to up the ante. *If you always do what you've always done, you'll always get what you always got.*

Meaning – if you want to look and feel fitter you need to do more than you are already doing. So if you're happy with your fitness level then fine, keep running round after the kids, but if you're looking to make improvements you have to increase to your activity levels.

If you want to improve your fitness levels rather than just maintain what you have, you need to up the ante.

Social Life

My friend couldn't come with me

Was your friend going to do your workout for you too?

I want to go to the pub instead

Being fit doesn't mean that you can't go to the pub. But it does mean that you can't go to the pub every time you get invited, and that you can't make the pub a priority over exercise. At least three times a week you *have* to make your workout the priority. So plan your weeks accordingly – get the workouts in your diary, and if you're invited for an impromptu drink after work on a workout day, you can say you have a prior engagement.

What do you want more? A fit healthy, attractive body and an occasional night at the pub, or a beer belly and a busy but unhealthy social life?

See also "I'm hungover" in the Body section

My friends say it's rubbish

And what was your opinion? Did you try it, or did you let someone else put you off? We're all different, with different strengths, weaknesses, likes and dislikes. Your friends may be carnivores, you may be a veggie. Your friends might like the theatre, you may prefer the cinema. That's just the way it is. Different things work for different people. So don't dismiss anything unless you've tried it yourself.

My boyfriend/girlfriend/spouse wants me to stay in

Aww! How sweet. And how flattering. But what do *you* want to do? How are you going to achieve your fitness goals if you don't do your workout? If you went and did it right now, wouldn't you be back in time to have some quality time together afterwards?

Feeling fitter will make you feel happier, more positive and nicer to be around.

When you're working towards a goal it's important to have people around you who support what you are doing, and who won't actively de-rail your efforts. For the future, have a chat to your partner. Explain that you'd like their support. Explain that feeling fitter will make you feel happier, more positive and nicer to be around. And you'll look good. That's the pay-off for them.

It's my friend/colleague/ relative's birthday/leaving do

Yes…but it's not YOUR party/leaving do!

There's no harm in having the occasional big (for "big" read "boozy") night out, but if you're serious about fitness you need to pick your occasions, and limit them. You don't have to accept every invitation you get.

If you really have to go on a night out, how about fitting in a workout beforehand – if everyone goes down the pub at 5.30, you can leave at the same time, get to the gym, get showered and be in the pub or restaurant by 7.30 – they'll all still be there. And then you have less drinking time too.

See also "I'm hungover" under Body.

I want to watch Eastenders/ TOWIE/etc

Ever heard of catch up TV?

Finances

Gym memberships are too expensive

Yes, some gyms are really expensive but the majority these days are reasonably priced, and if you shop around, consider taking an off-peak membership, wait for special offers to come up, or (if you're brave enough) try to negotiate a discount or a waiver of the joining fee, you might find you can stretch to the cost.

If you're really strapped for cash, struggling to make ends meet, and can't afford to join even a moderately priced gym, you can exercise for free outdoors or at home. Running is free, as is cycling if you already own a bike (or could borrow one). Try bodyweight exercises in your garden/home – try press-ups, squats, lunges, ab curls, planks, jumping jacks, burpees. Or buy a skipping rope. Get on YouTube and search for "home workouts" for an endless supply of free ideas.

If, however, you're earning a fair salary, but always have nothing left at the end of the month, consider keeping a money diary for a month – record everything you spend, right down to bottles of water, newspapers, gum. You might identify a small but regular expense which really adds up in the space of a month and which you could forego – daily coffee on the way to work anyone?

Also, look at your money diary to assess your priorities. Let's say a gym membership costs £55 per month. Sounds like a lot if you have zero left in your bank account at the end of every month. But what do you spend £55 on? A pair of shoes you didn't really need but just loved? Two bottles of wine and some bar snacks on a night out? A beauty treatment? What could you do without, or buy less often or find a cheaper alternative for that would save you enough for that gym membership?'

You can exercise for free outdoors or at home.

One final thought – the most expensive gym memberships are those which are never used. So if you do have one, make sure you get the most value from it by going often!

Location

I'm on holiday

This could be one of the few valid excuses in this book – alongside "I'm injured" and "I think I may be getting ill". Sometimes you just need to take a break. Holidays are all about cutting yourself some slack and taking a break from your usual routine. So if you normally exercise regularly and you're going on a short break (a week or less) then a few days of inactivity is not going to do too much damage – don't beat yourself up for taking a rest. What tends to do more damage is the holiday diet – alcohol every day, buffet breakfasts, cream teas, eating out every evening, ice creams between meals.

Before your holiday, decide how much slack you're going to allow yourself when you're away. What matters most to you? Taking a rest from physical activity or returning home as fit as you went away? If you want to maintain your fitness levels while you're away have a think about how much exercise you will need to do, plan how you're going to do it and take the necessary kit. And consider diarising the workouts, as it's easier than ever on holiday to say "I'll do it tomorrow", when you're feeling sluggish from too much food and alcohol.

But a holiday is a holiday – it's meant to be a break from your normal routine, so don't beat yourself up if you want complete relaxation – it's worth repeating that weight wise it's generally the holiday eating and drinking which does the damage, not the drop in activity levels.

The gym is too far away

If your journey to the gym is inconvenient, you're going to struggle to feel enthusiastic about going. The journey might also cost money you'd rather not spend in extra bus or train fares, or extra petrol for your car.

Unless you can adapt your daily routine (eg. keep your kit in your car and go on the way to or from work rather than getting home and then going out again), you're going to have to make a decision. Keep beating yourself up about not going to a gym that's too far away, or find a more convenient place to exercise.

If may be that you joined this particular gym because it was the best in the area. But what's more effective – belonging to a fantastic gym which you never travel to, or belonging to an adequate gym which you do visit as it's convenient?

Now I appreciate that city dwellers generally have a choice of local gyms, whereas if you live in the country you might not have a lot of choice. So if you can't make it to a gym at all, think about other forms of exercise or activity. If you can afford it, think about booking a person-

Make exercise as convenient as possible and you're far more likely to do it.

al trainer, or buy some equipment for your home. Make exercise as convenient as possible and you're far more likely to do it.

I travel a lot for work

In a previous life I used to do a lot of business travel. Where possible I would stay in a hotel with a gym. Generally the quality of hotel gyms is way below what you'd get at your own gym, but I've never been to one where I couldn't put together a workout of some sort. Yes, you have to take your kit with you, but a lightweight pair of trainers and some shorts and a tee shirt doesn't take up a lot of room in your suitcase.

If you don't have the option of staying in a hotel with a gym, try researching the area in which you'll be staying before you go, to see if there are any pay-as-you go gyms you could use.

And if you're completely stuck for a gym, think about what you can do in your hotel room – there is a wide range of body weight exercises which require no equipment – for instance, squats, lunges, crunches, press ups, burpees, planks. And if the area in which you're staying is safe, you can always go for a run.

My top tip is to invest in a resistance band, which takes up no weight in your suitcase but opens up a whole range of exercises you can do in your room – bicep curls, shoulder presses, rows, chest presses, tricep extensions. I used to take a band with me wherever I travelled for work. You'll find them on Amazon for a few pounds.

This is all pretty obvious stuff, but the key message is that you need to plan ahead – if you embark on your trip with no kit, no resistance band and no clue as to whether you'll have access to a gym at your destination, you're doomed before you get there.

Of course there is another element of business travel, which is the social element. It may be that you have hosts at your destination who feel obliged to entertain you every night – "entertainment" generally meaning too much food and too much alcohol. If you enjoy this, and look forward to it, then chances are you're not going to prioritise workouts! But if the socialising feels like part of the job and you'd rather not be doing quite so much of it, practice some polite responses to invitations in advance, or email your hosts in advance with reasons why you need some time alone in the evenings. If I was limited to doing workouts in my room, I always felt a bit embarrassed to admit this to clients so I would say I had some work to do or that I had to catch up on my emails or that I had a Skype call to make. If I was able to use the hotel gym, I would simply say I wanted to do a workout. Say it firmly and politely, don't waver and your hosts will respect your decision. They might even feel relieved that they don't have to spend their own leisure time entertaining you.

Logistics

My iPOD needs charging and I don't like to exercise without music

Hmmm, it may need charging now, but what plans do have in place generally to make sure all of the kit you need to have around you is charged, washed, packed and ready to go?

And as for today's session, how hard is it going to be to exercise without it? Or do you have a partner who'd let you borrow theirs? Or could you put it on charge for a few minutes while you change into your kit?

It's January and the gym's too busy

If you've made a new year's resolution to get fit and you've decided to do that by joining a gym, then you'll have to put up with the crowds of people just like you for a few weeks. But console yourself with the fact that if you stick with it, the gym will be much quieter by Easter! Not everyone will stick with it.

Most gyms offer special discounts and freebies in January, so you should be able to bag yourself a good deal, which might go some way to compensating for the crowds.

And get organised – if classes get full, you can often book in advance, which has the advantage of committing you to going.

You could also join the gym in advance of your resolution, in November or December. This gives you the chance to familiarise yourself with the layout and equipment, get your induction sessions done before the rush when staff have more time for you, and start establishing the habit of being there so that when the crowds do descend you're clear on what you're doing, aren't distracted and know which equipment is available as a backup if your first choice isn't available. This approach may have an added advantage helping to minimise the damage done by the Christmas excesses too!

I forgot my kit

I know someone who turned up to the gym one evening and realised she'd forgotten her leggings, gym bra and top – she had only trainers and socks. She wanted to work out so much that she bought a whole new outfit from the gym shop. Yes, she was loaded (or if you prefer, had more money than sense) and could afford to do this, and I appreciate that not everyone can, but she really did want to do that workout.

> When you fly off on holiday, do you ever forget your passport?

I also know someone who forgot his trainers and asked to rummage through the gym's lost property box to find a pair of trainers in his size – again, not a solution for everyone, particularly hygiene enthusiasts, but he really wanted to do his workout too.

If neither of those options appeals, and you really don't want to miss your workouts, the solution is to ensure that you never forget your kit again. How can you do that? Well, when you fly off on holiday, do you ever forget your passport? Or the last time you had tickets for a gig did you leave them on the kitchen table when you left the house? I am guessing not. Those things were so important to you that you made absolutely sure you remembered to take them with you – perhaps you stuck a post-it note on your fridge, or put a reminder on your phone, or located your passport a few days before and put it somewhere close to hand. Do you do any of these things to remind you about your kit?

Or how about a contingency plan? If you go to the gym after work, how about having a spare set of kit in the office or the boot of your car?

If you care enough about something you will ensure that everything is in place to make it happen.

Time

I don't have the time to exercise

Fetch a piece of paper and a pen. Write down how you spend a typical day – getting up, showering, watching TV, checking Facebook and Twitter, chatting, reading magazines, painting your nails, gaming…?   Most people waste time every day without realising it.

If you're truly time poor (you've got young kids or elderly parents to care for, or work really long hours), have a think about how you can make your chosen form of exercise as efficient as possible. Try a High Intensity Interval Training (HIIT) version of what you usually do – if you normally run for an hour, do 20 minutes of intervals. The deal with HIIT is that the intense segments need to be all-out effort, but you save time and it's extremely efficient for improving fitness and burning fat. Look it up on the internet and you'll find lots of ideas and sample workouts.

If you don't have the time to go to the gym because it takes too long to travel there, see "The gym is too far away" under Location.

Can you combine your workouts with other activities? Perhaps do a class with a friend instead of going to the cinema? Go for a walk with a friend rather than a coffee?

Review your Benefits List, remind yourself how much you want to get fit, and *create* and diarise the time you need for your workouts. And check that when you do exercise, you are exercising in the most optimal way – ask advice from a seasoned runner, a personal trainer, or your class instructor. When your time is precious it's important to use it as wisely as possible.

> When your time is precious it's important to use it as wisely as possible.

I'll start again on Monday

This one generally works in conjunction with another excuse. You've probably already missed one workout, let's say Tuesday's run, using one of the other excuses listed in this book. You get home on Wednesday, tired from a hard day's work, and you decide you'll start running again next week.

This is very similar to dieters who have a healthy

breakfast, a healthy lunch, then follow the healthy lunch with a cake. Then they say they'll start the diet again tomorrow. One piece of cake would not have had much of an effect on their weight loss. But the

You need to have a plan!

second piece, the Coke mid-afternoon, the takeaway in the evening and the multiple glasses of wine to wash it down definitely will. One slip shouldn't be allowed to turn into a major slide.

So, one skipped session is not going to make a massive difference as long as it is just *one* skipped session. The missed run on a Tuesday wouldn't hurt too much if you'd gone out on Wednesday instead and then got back to normal, but a missed run on a Tuesday followed by inactivity on Wednesday, Thursday, Friday, Saturday and Sunday isn't serving your plans to get fitter.

So if you are reading this with your mind set on missing a session now, and you've already missed a session this week, consider what you're actually contemplating – you are planning to miss two, three, maybe four of your planned sessions. And if you're thinking "What you do you mean 'planned' sessions?" take a look at "I don't have time" in the Time section – you need to have a plan!

I've got chores to do

No one ever lay on their death bed wishing they'd done more cleaning. But I'm sure quite a few people lay there wishing they'd taken more care of their health.

Of course chores need to be done – if you never washed up or loaded the dishwasher you'd have no plates on which to serve your healthy meals – but there might be some things which don't need to be done quite so often or quite so rigorously. So it just comes down to a question of priorities – do you really need to clean the windows weekly or could you do it fortnightly or monthly and free up some time to exercise?

If you're not short of cash could you pay someone else to do the cleaning/gardening/take the dog for a walk? If you have young kids, can you offer extra pocket money in exchange for doing chores? What else could you do to reduce the amount of time you spend on chores?

I need to look after the kids

I appreciate that you have responsibilities. Being a parent takes up an enormous amount of time and it's often probably your top priority. If your kids are very small, sleep may well be your top priority.

But as explained in "I don't have the energy to exercise", getting fitter will give you more energy, and this in turn will help you to cope with the demands of being a parent. If you are slumping exhausted on the sofa every evening after bedtime, possibly with a glass of wine and/or a food treat, due to being tired out by keeping up with your young family, you might find that fitting in some exercise will help you cope better with the stress involved in having a packed family diary, and generally improve your mood.

Exercise will help you cope better with the stress involved in having a packed family diary.

Of course you probably already know this, and you're looking into your over-filled diary and struggling to see how you can fit workouts in. So how about exercising *with* your children? There are lots of activities for families to do together – cycling, swimming or walking for instance. Try making it fun by playing old school games – skipping, hopscotch, chase, or go to an adventure playground. Great fun for children of all ages!

And finally – do you want your children to grow up fit and active? If so, what better way to encourage them than to set an example?

The Lamest Excuses of All

I got home from work, sat down on the sofa and couldn't get up again

Really? Not to go to the toilet? Or fetch a snack? Or go to bed? Or is your sofa made of very strong Velcro?

Are you are actually saying "I got home from work, sat down on the sofa and made the decision that I would skip my workout tonight"? The sofa did not make that decision for you, even if it is a really comfortable one.

See also "I don't have the energy to exercise" in the Body section.

I hate my gym

So why are you still a member?!

What is it you hate? If it's the general atmosphere, you might want to try another gym where you feel more comfortable – every gym is different, with different types of members, different equipment and classes, and different corporate images. Even two gyms in the same chain will differ according to their location.

But is it the gym you hate, or something else? If you hate exercising in public, see "I don't want to look stupid" in the Mind section of this book. If you hate the forms of exercise on offer, try something new outside of a gym. If you don't enjoy the exercise, see "It's no fun", also in Mind.

Every gym is different.

And remember that getting fit is always going to require *some* effort – if getting fit was easy, everyone would be super fit. If you want it enough you're going to have to work for it.

It will mess up my hair

Yes it most definitely will, if done with enough gusto. That's why gyms have showers, hair dryers, etc. Build in time after your workout to deal with your hair. Sorted.

I can't get out of bed in the morning

I'm not sure this is actually true – I am guessing that you *do* get out of bed every morning at some point – to go to work, to eat breakfast, to get on with your day?

So what you're saying is not that you are stuck in your bed but that you don't want to get out of bed early enough to do an early morning workout. The simple answer? Work out later in the day.

Exercise at the start of the day is energising.

But if you like the idea of doing your workout first thing, you have to develop a habit of getting up early, so that getting up at 6.00am to do your workout becomes as normal as getting up at 7.00am to go to work.

In preparation for this, ask yourself why you want to do this – what advantages do early morning workouts have over evening/daytime workouts? I'll start you off – exercise at the start of the day is energising, it means you're in no danger of skipping it if you have a hard day at work, it leaves your evenings free to do other things, and it's generally easier to schedule – excluding child care, most people don't have other commit-

Try gently easing yourself into early starts.

ments to juggle at 6.30 in the morning. As always, re-mind yourself of the benefits of what you want to do to motivate yourself to get on and do it.

Try gently easing yourself into early starts – next week, plan to get up early on just one day. When the alarm goes off, tell yourself it's just one day, and that to-morrow and all the other days of the week you can lay in bed for longer. Make this one day a fixed day every week, and stick to it for a month. The following month, add another early start into your week and go with two early workouts a week for another month.

Then you can take a view on whether you want to increase these early starts, or whether you can really only deal with two per week. You don't have to do ev-ery workout first thing.

Some Final Thoughts

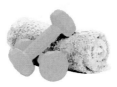

You'll never regret a workout. Every workout is one step closer to where you want to be – that leaner, fitter, stronger body, that feeling of wellbeing, and every single item on your Benefits List.

When you're considering skipping a workout, take a few minutes to remind yourself why you decided to get fit in the first place. And how will you feel in an hour's time if you haven't done it? Do you really want to feel that? And how will you feel in an hour's time if you *have* done it?

When you start to tackle your excuses and start to exercise more regularly, you're forming habits which will eventually become part of your life.

> Every workout is one step closer to where you want to be.

Prioritise your workouts and plan your life around them, just like you'd prioritise anything which is important to you. If you're aiming at a reasonable 3-4 workouts a week you only need to find 6-8 hours a week (I'm including some showering/travel time). That's less than 5% of your week, or 7% of your waking hours.

And plan, plan plan! Without planning, things go awry. Let's say you want to fit in three workouts in a week, but you don't plan exactly when. Monday night comes along and you've got that Monday feeling, so you say to yourself you'll go to the gym tomorrow. But you then realise you're meeting friends on Tuesday, which means no workout, and you're going away at the weekend, so opportunities to fit in your three workouts are disappearing fast. If you'd looked ahead and diarised those workouts, you'd not get halfway through the week and realise you'd lost your opportunities.

Prioritise your workouts and plan your life around them.

With a little planning, you can build your own contingency plans, and prepare to overcome obstacles. Spend an hour every Sunday diarising workouts for the coming week, wash your gym kit and charge your iPod. These things will make a big difference to how likely you are to succeed.

It's also really important to set clear goals and record your progress. There's a well-worn motivational quote which says "If you don't know where you are going, you'll end up somewhere else". You need to know exactly what you are aiming at, and by when, so that you can put a plan together. You want to be fitter, but how much fitter? In three/six/twelve months' time, what do you want to be able to do? Run a marathon, or run in a 5k charity run? Be selected for the local football team, or be fit enough to knock a ball around the park with your grandkids? Look better on the beach or compete in a CrossFit competition?

When my clients describe their goals to me, the two questions I ask are "By when do you want to achieve this?" and "How will you know when you have achieved it?"

So set a date – without a deadline you'll drift. What's another day of not working towards your goal if there is no date by which you have to achieve it? *Set a date*.

> Without a deadline you'll drift.

Then be very specific about what it is you want to achieve. For instance, how many inches will you have lost or how many kilos will you have dropped in order to say "I've lost weight"? How many press-ups do you want to be able to do before you can say "I've got stronger"? *Write it down.*

Using the current state of affairs as your starting point with your documented, specific end point, you can now chart your progress. Think about creating some sort of journal or spreadsheet or download an app which you can use to record progress. You may only be recording small improvements, but those small improvements will add up to one great big improvement if you stick at it. Aim for a small improvement every time you work out – one more minute, one more rep, one more kilogram, a little bit faster, a little less rest. And if you ever feel disheartened, you can look back on your progress to date. Measure, record and time your way to success.

You can actually get pretty fit in less time than you think – if you know what to do. So if you can afford it, consider getting a personal trainer or expert coach and use him/her properly: that is, not to motivate you to turn up to the gym or sports ground (that's your own job!) but to advise and educate you on the most effective way to exercise when you are there. Ask for recommendations and get a good one. A few sessions could be all you need to get on the right track.

Finally, make sure you do something you enjoy. You won't stick with something which bores you. And be aware that you could learn to love the really hard stuff if you stick with it long enough to see results.

Make sure you do something you enjoy.

If you've never been particularly fit it might take you a while to change the way you see yourself. At 40 I still saw myself as the gawky kid at school who couldn't catch a ball and was last to be picked for teams. I'm almost 50 now but after getting some good advice, learning to exercise effectively and sticking with it I'm finally able to accept that I am a Fit Person (most of the time). You too will become a Fit Person if you keep at it.

Exercise is a lifelong commitment but feeling fit and strong will improve EVERYTHING about your life. It gave me the confidence to leave a job I hated and set up two businesses.

So prioritise and plan your workouts, make it as easy as possible for yourself, form the habit and reap the benefits – it *will* be worth it.

And no more excuses!

I'd love to hear from you if this book has helped you, or if you have an excuse which I have missed! You can email me at joanne@joannehenson.co.uk.

Acknowledgements

I'd like to say a big thank you to the following individuals:

Gill Williams for proof reading and editing the original version of this book

Jeremy Boyd, Paul Stevenson and Ben Peel for their expert advice and killer workouts, and for ensuring that I never feel the need to use an excuse to skip a workout

My partner Andy for patiently listening to all of my ideas for this book and others, when he'd rather have been listening to Led Zeppelin

Reference/ Bibliography

MARTHA BECK *The 4-Day Win: Change the way you think about food and your body in just 4 days*
Piatkus, 2008

PAUL DOLAN *Happiness by Design: Finding Pleasure and Purpose in Everyday Life*
Allen Lane, 2014

ELISABETH WILSON *Stress Proof Your Life: 52 Brilliant Ideas for Taking Control*
Infinite Ideas, 2007

Index

Also in this series

What's Your Excuse for not Eating Healthily?

Joanne Henson
***Overcome your excuses and eat well to look good
and feel great***

Do you wish you could eat more healthily and improve
the way you look and feel, but find that all too often life
gets in the way? Do you regularly embark on healthy
eating plans or diets but find that you just can't stick
with them? Then this is the book for you.

This isn't another diet book. Instead it's a look at the
things which have tripped you up in the past and offers advice, ideas and inspiration to help you overcome
those things this time around.

No willpower? Hate healthy food? Got no time to
cook? Crave sugary snacks? Overcome all of these excuses and many more. Change your eating habits and
relationship with food *for good*.

"Very useful, very practical and makes a lot of sense!

There are some great tips in here and even if you just implemented a bit of Joanne's advice it would make a real difference"

Chantal Cooke, journalist & broadcaster

Paperback – ISBN 978-0-9933388-2-3
e-book – ISBN 978-0-9933388-3-0

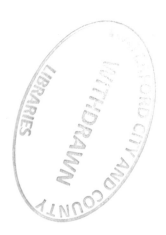

Also in this series

What's Your Excuse for not Living a Life You Love?

Monica Castenetto
Overcome your excuses and lead a happier, more fulfilling life

Are you stuck in a life you don't love? Have you reached a point where your life doesn't feel right for you any-more? Then this book is for you.

This is not yet another self-help book claiming to re-veal the secret to permanent happiness. Instead, it helps you to tackle the things which have been holding you back and gives ideas, advice and inspiration to help you move on to a better life.

Don't know what you want? Scared of failure? Hate change? Worried about what others might think? This book will help you overcome all of your excuses and give you the motivation you need to change your life.

"Monica's energy, enthusiasm for life and her grounded, supportive coaching style never fail to

stimulate and inspire her clients to find ways to live a life they love"

Nicci Bonfanti, Master Trainer and Coach

Paperback – ISBN 978-0-9933388-4-7
e-book – ISBN 978-0-9933388-5-4